# Essential Oils for Babies

*(The Definitive Guide)*

*Essential Oils For Your Baby's Heath, Vitality and Longevity*

# Table of Contents

# Introduction

Being a parent is one of the best jobs in the world but it is also one of the hardest. We want our kids to have the best of everything, from the day they are born until the day that they die. In the modern world, figuring out what is best for our family can be tough - we keep reading about how much there is out there to be worried about in terms of the the chemicals being used in the processing and manufacturing of food, toys, medicine and even clothing.

It can seem like a veritable minefield as there is much debate over these issues - some experts believe, for example, that a low-fat diet is the way to stay healthy, some believe that cutting out carbohydrates is the way to go and that is only one of the many debates.

The one thing that the experts do seem to agree on, however, is that we should be looking for ways to simplify our lives and live lives that are more in tune with the natural order. All the experts agree that heavily processed and refined foods should be kept to a bare minimum.

In terms of lifestyle, experts also agree that we should be living simpler lives, reducing stress and the amounts of chemicals that we expose our bodies to. A simpler life, with fewer chemicals is something that resonates within many of us and so it has been one that is eagerly adopted.

The first step, naturally is to look at your diet and lifestyle. The next step, especially if you have just had a baby, is to look at decreasing the amounts of chemicals in your home.

According to a study conducted in Canada, a direct link was found between the lack of diversity when it came to the bacteria in the gut and the increased potential for developing food allergies at the age of 12 months. The study points to a very real problem when it comes to infants - the use of antibiotics early in life can lead to upsets in the digestive flora and so could increase the chances of the child developing allergies and food sensitivities.

Whilst the researchers do state that there is more work to be done, the study does give pause for thought - why take a chance unless it is absolutely necessary? Are there even alternatives?

The great news is that, as you will see in this book, you can take very real steps to improving baby's health and well-being without needing to rely on conventional medicine that can damage their delicate systems.

This book will guide you through the use of essential oils on a day to day basis to boost your baby's immunity, help him sleep better, keep him calm and relaxed and healthy.

# Chapter 1: Why You Should Use Essential Oils for Your Baby

## A Naturally Good, Safe Remedy

The "all-natural" bandwagon is not a new one but it now seems that it is really gaining traction in our society now, instead of being viewed as a "kooky" remedy. There is now a plethora of information out there about complimentary therapies that you can use for your family and yourself.

I am not here to knock conventional medicine - conventional medicine performs a vital role in some cases - I am just suggesting adopting a more gentle approach. An approach that works in harmony with your system, without the use of synthetic drugs and compounds.

Aromatherapy ticks all of the boxes when it comes to a wholly natural therapy and there is nothing "new age" about it. Essential oils have been used for thousands of years as a valid and useful form of treatment. Scientists studying these oils have found that they do indeed have healing properties and are, in some cases, as effective or more effective than traditional medication.

In fact, some of the oils are so complex in structure that we are not even able to copy them in the most advanced laboratories.

I started experimenting with aromatherapy when my eldest daughter was 7 months old. She had an infection and the doctor prescribed antibiotics. She reacted badly to the antibiotics and came quite close to death - as it turned out, she was allergic to the medication.

After that scare, I decided that there had to be a better way. I didn't want my child to ever need to take conventional medicine again so I started reading up on alternative treatments. The treatment option that resonated best with me was aromatherapy so I read up on it and was hooked from that day forward.

It was the best move I could have possibly made as a parent and I am pleased to say that my kids, even now that they are grown, seldom need to see a doctor.

It still amazes me that one little bottle of oil contains the potential for healing a wide range of conditions. I also like how easy the oils are to use. You can pop some in the bath, add them to a cold/ warm compress, add them to some oil or cream, diffuse them or even just put them on a tissue and sniff at them that way. I even, from time to time, pick up a bottle of one of my favorite oils and take a huge whiff. Whether you need to calm down or need to gear up, the oils can help you.

I feel that they helped me be a better, and more patient parent to my kids. The primary benefit, however, was to my kids themselves - once I had built up a small arsenal of essential oils, I found that I had everything that I needed to help them with the little bumps, bruises and childhood illnesses that every kid has to face.

With my second-eldest child, John, I started using essential oils much earlier than I had with the first and the results were really amazing. John suffered from eczema from early on and it really caused him a lot of discomfort.

Fortunately, as soon as he was old enough, I mixed up a batch of cream to help him. It took a bit of tweaking but, before long, I was largely able to get rid of his eczema. An adult now, he does have the occasional flare-up, especially when he is under pressure, but I just mix up a batch of the cream for him and it sorts it out quite quickly.

If you, like me, are worried about the effect of the long-term use of conventional medication will have on your baby, or, if you just want an alternative that is as effective without nasty side effects, essential oils are an avenue worth exploring.

Give it a try - I will give you plenty of information on how to get started, the oils that you will use and the conditions that can be treated. You will learn how to safely use the oils and I am sure that you will have a lot of fun in the process.

## Using This Book

You do not have to read this book from cover to cover in order to get the information that you need but I do urge you to thoroughly read Chapters 2-4 very carefully before starting out.

Essential oils are a natural treatment but also a very powerful one. You need no more than a few drops of any oil at a time. I cover the proper dilution of the oils in Chapter 4. In Chapter 2, you will be given important safety hints so be sure to read through this chapter carefully.

Chapter 3 will be useful when it comes to choosing the oils that you will use. There are hundred of oils out there so I have narrowed the list down to the oils that I find most useful and have explained a little about each oil and what it does. There is also a list of common ailments and which oils are suitable to treat these at every age.

# Chapter 2: Safety Tips

## To Make Sure That You Get the Best Possible Results

Let us get to grips with the safety issues when it comes to using essential oils. Whilst this is a wholly natural treatment, it does pay to take some care in the application of the oils. The oils are highly concentrated and can irritate or burn the skin if not applied in the correct proportions.

Further to that, overuse can lead to a toxic buildup in the liver, especially in the case of very young children. The fact that the essential oils are made up of such potent compounds means that not all oils can be safely used for younger children.

Think of it this way - the essential oils are basically similar in nature to a herbal tea but about 1000 times more concentrated. The plants are put through a distiller and the essence that makes up the oils is extracted. It can take thousands of petals to produce even just one small bottle of oils.

If we go back to the herbal tea analogy, the equivalent would be to drink thousands of cups of tea in one go. (Except that you would never drink essential oils - they are far too concentrated).

Now, let's get down to the safety tips.

# Choose Quality

Aromatherapy is very popular and there are many companies out there that have now jumped on the bandwagon. Some of these companies deliver high quality products, others do not. Take, for example, the range of shampoos, aqueous creams, etc. that have essential oils added into them.

These products usually smell quite good and are nice to use but the truth is that the amount of essential oils used is negligible and, considering all the processing the product has undergone, not going to do you much good anyway. See for yourself - compare the smell of one of these products to the smell of pure essential oils and you will quickly notice a difference.

You are far better off making your own formulations using high quality oils to use on your baby.

The key is to find 100% pure oils, or oils marked "Therapeutic Grade". You cannot always get these in your local department store, you may have to visit a health store or look online for the right oils. It is worth taking some extra time in the beginning to source the best essential oils that you can afford  and doing so will pay off in a big way later on down the line.

You should never settle for cheap imitations, especially when you will be using these oils on your baby. You are best off dealing with a company that has an established, good reputation.

The problem with dealing with the cheapest brands is that you can never really be quite sure what went into the oils in the first place. Some essential oils, like Lavender, are easy to produce and so can be sold for less. Some oils, like Rose, are really expensive to produce and so it becomes expensive to offer the pure oil.

The less scrupulous companies will dilute the oil with an oil that is cheaper to produce. It will still smell pretty much the same, but you have no idea what you are getting. In addition, the oils that they start off with are bound to be low-quality in the first place and extracted in the quickest and easiest manner possible. In general, these companies are looking to make a quick buck and so you will often find that these cheaper oils have higher levels of solvents and other undesirable chemicals.

To quickly check whether you have the real deal or not, look for the words, "100% Pure" or "Therapeutic Grade". In addition to the common name, such as Melissa, the oils ought to have their botanical name, such as Melissa Officinalis on the bottle as well - this is standard for all therapeutic grade oils.

Companies many also choose to list the method of distillation and the region of origin for the oil.

## Where the Oil Originates

The components in an oil can from one season to the next and also from one region to the next. This is because of the climatic differences from one region to the next, even when plants of the same species are used. Even the soil that the plant has been grown in can make a difference to the components.

Still, this is not all that important, as long as you are dealing with a reputable company that sources the best materials and that ensures that high quality standards are maintained.

## The Extraction Process

Again, if you have stuck to a reputable provider, you do not need to worry about this as much. There are several ways to extract the essential oils and, to get the best results, the right extraction method is necessary. For example, when it comes to oils that are resinous in nature, or oils that are heat sensitive, solvent extraction is usually the best option.

Your more robust oils stand up well to the distillation process whereby the plants are subjected to high heat and pressure in order to extract the oils.

Why this matters to you is that the cheaper brands tend to have higher traces of solvent residue or may use methods of extraction that damage the actual component content of the oils in general. If they use high heat to distill Jasmine oil, for example, the oil will not fare well at all.

## Blended Oils

It is common practise to blend the more expensive oils such as Jasmine and Rose with less expensive counterparts in order to make the oils more affordable. This is not necessarily a bad thing - it can give you access to oils that you would not easily be able to afford otherwise.

As long as the company concerned is completely upfront about the oils used, there should be no problems because they will also tell you what oils were blended together. You then just need to check that those oils are suitable for use with babies.

At times, these blends can even prove more useful than the pure oil would have been on its own. Geranium essential oil is often blended with Rose as the scents and properties are similar and the blend on the whole has more powerful properties when it comes to skin rejuvenation.

If you find an oil that is marked "Rose Blend", for example, but there is no indication on the bottle of what oils were blended with the Rose oil, it is better not to buy it.

# You Get What you Pay For

This is very true when it comes to essential oils. You will be amazed to see how much the prices differ from range to range and you may well feel that the more expensive ranges are a rip off. It pays to remember, however, that you get what you pay for.

If a company is offering an essential oil that is a lot less expensive than its corresponding counter-parts in different ranges, then they must be cutting corners somewhere along the line - either by adulterating the oil or by using an inferior quality oil.

Also check what the price differences are between different oils in the same range. Roman Chamomile oil, for example, will be more expensive than Eucalyptus oil because the oil is more difficult to extract. If you find that all the prices within a specific range are around about the same, be careful - it is natural that some oils are more expensive than others and not normal for all the oils to be priced the same. If they are all the same price, it is probably an indication that they are adulterated or of a lower quality.

# I Hate Fragrance Oils

I don't know exactly when it happened but today air fresheners are the norm in many homes. When we were growing up, we didn't use these artificial sprays and I have become convinced that the higher levels of respiratory ailments in children can be as a result of using some of these products.

My absolute pet peeve is the use of Fragrance oils and I advise everyone against using them. They are completely artificial and every time you use them, you are introducing those artificial chemicals into the air.

If you must fragrance your home, use essential oils. A mixture of a cup of baking soda with a few drops of your favorite essential oil can be sprinkled over carpets in the home and then vacuumed up to lightly freshen the scent of the room.

In addition, fragrance oils really have no therapeutic properties at all and are best left on the shelf at the store.

## Dilution and Dilute Again

Essential oils that are going to come into contact with your baby's skin must be diluted. Because they are so concentrated, there is a very real danger of them irritating or burning your baby's skin when they are applied neat or in high concentrations. Sensitization may also develop when the oils are too strong. Whilst there is a lot of information out there that says that it is okay to apply Lavender oil and Tea Tree oil neat, I advise against doing this until your child is at least two years old.

As a general rule, until your baby turns two, you should never use any oils neat on his skin. What is actually great about this is that the oils, even diluted at 0.5% will still get the job done. The blend may not smell very strong to you but it will be perfect for baby. Babies are a lot smaller in size than adults so you should never use the same concentration of oils on them that you would on yourself.

If you are concerned about the time factor in blending up the oils as and when you need them, just make up a bottle to keep at the ready. In my house, I always keep a blend of Lavender oil - it is used often to soothe rashes, headaches, sunburn, etc.

For more on how to properly dilute the oils, refer to Chapter 4.

# Keep the Oils Locked Away

Little kids are very curious and are very good at getting into places that they should not. Little fingers are more adept at opening bottles that you may realize and essential oil bottles are not child safe.

It is best to keep the oils under lock and key until your child is old enough to understand that they should not mess with them. If you don't, your child may take it into his head to apply the oils, a potentially painful experience or drink the oils, a potentially deadly experience.

If your child does manage to get into your essential oils and use them, be sure to clean away any residue from the skin as quickly as possible. A damp cloth will do the trick. Immediately apply a plain aqueous cream to calm any irritation. If the skin does burn, get the child to the doctor.

If the oils get into his eyes, rinse the eyes with plain milk as quickly as possible. Repeat until the stinging stops. Water is not advisable here as it will not neutralize the oils. Act quickly to prevent permanent damage. Don't let your child rub their eyes as this will make things worse.

If your child swallows the oils, try to get them to throw up and then go straight to the emergency room.

# Ingesting the Oils

In French aromatherapy, there is a branch of therapy that centers around taking the oils internally. This is not common practice here in the States and I advise against it - for adults and children. In France, the oils are only taken internally under the supervision of a licensed professional. This is not a practice that you should ever adopt at home as the oils can be potentially deadly when taken in the wrong quantities.

Eucalyptus, for example, a fatal dose may be as little as 4ml.

Besides which, the inhalation of the oils through the lungs or the absorption through the skin is a much more effective delivery method anyway. If you take the oils internally, you will have to wait until they have passed out of the stomach and into the digestive tract before absorption can commence. In addition, the stomach acid may damage some of the more sensitive components within the oil.

# NO Oils for Newborns

You should never use essential oils on a baby that is less than 10-12 weeks of age. In this critical stage just after birth, their systems are not yet equipped to dealing with the properties of the oils and you could risk them becoming sensitized to the oils that you use.

Extend this period if your baby was born prematurely to 10-12 weeks of the expected due date.

At this critical stage, the detoxifying effects of the essential oils may be too much for your child to handle.

Once they are over 10 weeks old, you may start using Lavender and Chamomile oils - both of which are gentle and soothing. Before covering your baby's body with either oil, you need to test a small amount on the skin to make sure that there is no allergic reaction.

If you are going to use a diffuser, you should start in a room that is fairly well-ventilated and add only a drop or two of the oil to be diffused. Watch baby carefully for any signs of distress - labored breathing or upset - to ensure that he is not allergic to the oils being diffused.

If you do notice problems, switch off the diffuser immediately and move your baby to another room.

## Small Child, Small Dose

When dosing your baby with cough syrup, would you ever give them the same amount that you yourself would take? The same principle applies when you are using essential oils - the smaller the child, the lower the dose and concentration of the oils needs to be.

One area that I find people make mistakes with is when it comes to different blends. The maximum dose for a 12 week old baby, for example, is 1 drop for every 10ml of oil. Most people easily get this right when using just one oil. Where they slip up is when it comes to adding the second and third oil - they increase the concentration without realizing it by adding in extra drops of oil. To avoid making the same mistake, always ensure that you add 10ml of carrier oil for every single drop of essential oil.

You can learn more about the correct dosages in Chapter 4.

# Oils that Cause Sensitivity to Light

Not all oils react well to the sun. When these oils are exposed to the light, they cause a reaction in the skin. This could lead to skin discoloration or irritation. Citrus oils are the oils most likely to react in this manner to the sun. My advice is to ensure that you only apply these oils when it is dark or that you ensure that your child is not exposed to sunlight for at least an hour or two after you have applied the oils.

# Careful Storage Required

Essential oils vary in stability from oils that are highly volatile, such as Jasmine, to oils that are very stable, such as Sandalwood. In order to extend the useful life of the oils, you need to make sure that you store them properly.

They need to be kept in a cool, dark place - exposure to heat and sunlight will have a negative effect on their longevity.

The same can be said for the carrier oils that you will use.

It may seem to make sense to store them in the kitchen or the bathroom but I advise  against this because these two rooms are the ones most likely to be affected by heat and moisture.

If you have made up blends of oils, the same rules apply to their storage as well.

When you are finished with the oil, the carrier oils or your blends, be sure to close the lids snugly as many of the oils can be subject to oxidization and  could evaporate if not closed properly after use.

# Checking the Oils for Rancidity

Essential oils will expire in time. As they age, they start to lose potency and will eventually degrade. In some oils, like citrus oils, this process is quicker than in others, like Sandalwood. The more volatile oils will typically be okay for about 6 months and the more stable ones could last a couple of years. If the oil smells odd or has sediments in it, it is best thrown out as it has gone off. The quality of the oil that you buy and how well it has been stored will also impact the longevity of the oil.

The best advice when it comes to essential oils is to only buy the amount that you can use within a 6 month period. Rather buy fewer bottles of oil and have less variety than having to throw out a whole lot of oils that have gone off. The bottles are not that big but 1 drop of oil is about the equivalent of half a milliliter so that one bottle does go quite far.

The same advice applies to the carrier oils that you buy. I would advise buying only as much as you would use in a 6 month period. With the special treatment oils you need to be especially careful as you will not use as much of them as you would your normal base oil or aqueous cream. I never buy more than 100ml - 250ml special treatment oils at the same time.

Sweet Almond oil and Grape Seed oil, on the other hand, have a much longer life span and are much more stable. If you plan to give baby a daily massage or incorporate the oils into your own regime, it is more economical to buy a liter bottle of these if you can. Both Sweet Almond and Grape Seed oil can be safely stored for a year or two, under optimal conditions.

Blends should also come into this category. You can improve the shelf life of a blend by adding in oils that have fixative properties -

Cedar Wood and Sandalwood oils are prime examples of this. These stable oils bind with the more volatile oils and help to stave off oxidization. Your blend, if stored properly, could last up to a year or so.

In all cases, it is a good idea to be wary of oils that have changed texture, color or aroma or that have got sediments in the bottom.

It may seem wasteful but it is best to throw away oils that you are not sure of - rancid oils can seriously irritate baby's skin and cause him to get sick.

## Simple is Better

When I started learning about essential oils, I was very anxious to get the full benefits and wanted to skip ahead to the blending - I reasoned that if one oil was good, three or four oils were even better. I ended up making some really awful mixtures.

Not all oils are compatible with one another and these oils, if blended together, create a blend that is bland and uninteresting or that really does not smell good. If you want to experiment, try mixing Lavender oil with Lemon oil. This will give you an idea of a disharmonious blend of oils. These blends score poorly in the scent department and fare even better when it comes to their medicinal benefits. The oils will actually work against one another so you won't get any benefit from them at all.

When mixing oils for your baby, simpler is better - you don't want to assail their senses with a myriad of smells. I advise first using each individual oil on its own so that you know what your baby likes and dislikes and whether or not there are any health issues to consider as well.

Once you know what oils you can safely use, then you can start trying to blend them. I suggest that you mix two oils at a time until you get used to blending. With babies, you should rather use less oils in a blend. I would usually advocate no more than three oils at a time.

I also believe that everyone who uses essential oils needs to get themselves a good overall guide that details the properties of each oil, its components, which oils it blends with, etc. You will find yourself often referring to your essential oil books so getting a good general encyclopedia is never a waste of time.

In general, oils of the same botanical family and oils that have similar compounds in them will blend well together. You will generally find that certain categories of oils will generally blend well with one another - spice and citrus oils are one great example of this, as are citrus and wood oils.

When you are starting out, look at the oils used in the blends that I have given you as a base for which oils blend well with others. Start out by making simple blends and gradually increase the number of oils used. Over time, you will be able to instinctively know a good blend from a bad one just by the scent.

As a general rule, stick to blends of three oils at most - event the most experienced blender has trouble distinguishing the different oils in such a blend. You can safely blend up to 5 oils but after that it becomes really complicated because you have to ensure that all the scents work well together and that all the oils blend well with each other as well.

You should also take note of what properties each oil has and try not to mix oils that have properties that are completely opposite. For example, Roman Chamomile is a sedative oil and Rosemary is a stimulant oil - they do not make a good blend.

# Write it Down

When I first started blending oils, I was cocky - I believed that I would always remember the blends that I had concocted and would always be able to tell one blend from another. Wrong!

It is not just the oils that you need to remember but also the exact quantities of each oil that makes a difference. Now you might be able to say, after a few weeks, which oil predominates a blend but you are unlikely to remember what proportions you used.

Why give yourself extra work? Get yourself a nice journal or notebook and write down the oils you have added to a blend, as soon as you have finished making the blend. As a busy parent, you have enough to keep track of so give yourself a break and make notes.

It can save you tons of time later when it comes to recreating the blends that worked well.

When I wised up, I got myself an A-4 hardcover notebook and started using it to record my efforts. Now, decades later, the book is looking a little worn but I refer to it whenever I need to whip up a batch of oils. It came in especially useful in writing this book as it jogged my memories for recipes that I used on my kids.

Write down the oils that you used and how much of each oil you used. Also make a note of what your first reaction was to the blend and how baby liked it. Also note down whether or not it worked well - this will help you to tweak the blends until you get them perfect. You will find over time that you come up with some tried and true recipes of your own that you will be able to use with all your kids and even your grand kids.

You are bound to find that your friends also want oils from you and so you need to keep track of which blends you gave to which friends in case they ask for a refill.

For me there is nothing more satisfying than finding a blend that works really well, and nothing quite as depressing as not being able to remember what you put into it.

## Basic Blending

I am going to cover some of the main points when it comes to blending but I do also urge you to do some research of your own. Learning to blend essential oils is a useful skill and once you have got the basics down, you can create an infinite number of blends.

I suggest starting out with only a small amount of your carrier oil so that you can get the scent right first and so that it is not as much of a big deal if you need to throw the blend out. Add in any special treatment oils once you have gotten the scent part right as these can be pricey and you don't want to waste them if you can avoid it.

The oils that you use are as much a matter of personal taste as a matter of choosing oils with the right properties. Add oils one drop at a time and smell in between each addition to check that you like the way that the scent of the blend is heading.

The base notes, for example, Sandalwood and Vertiver, have a much richer and more powerful scent and so you can get away with using smaller quantities of them to avoid them taking over your blend completely. Lavender oil is another example of an oil that has a strong scent - you may need to compensate by adding more of your other scents. A scent like Jasmine or Ylang Ylang can be quite heady out of the bottle but can help to tone down the heavier oils in a blend, adding a nice balanced quality to the oils.

Once you are satisfied with the scent of the blend, carefully check that the dilution is right for baby. In need, add more carrier oil in order to dilute the oils. Don't worry about this affecting the scent, it won't have much of an impact as the carrier oils take on the scent of any oil added to them.

I will deal with the right essential oils to use for your baby and what ages that the oils are suitable for in Chapter 3. My advice when it comes to young children is to avoid the more exotic blends as these can be over-powering and a baby is not able to communicate this to you.

## A Balanced Blend

It is nice to spend a bit more time on making a balanced scent when it comes to the oils, even if they are for your baby.

A balanced blend of oils is more pleasing to the senses and the smell of the blend can be as important in treating the mind as the physical compounds in the oil are in treating the body.

The basics are simple - always round off a blend with a high note, a middle note and a base note to make the blend more balanced. Jasmine and Neroli are good examples of high notes.

The high note is the aroma that is most volatile and that is smelt immediately when the oils are applied or diffused. It dissipates quite quickly leaving you with the middle note. Lavender and Chamomile are good examples of middle notes.

The middle note has a lot more body and a bit more staying power and will linger for about an hour or two. Sandalwood, Cedar Wood and Vertiver are good examples of base notes.

When blending for baby, I don't view it important to get in all the notes, especially if the baby is younger. I do think that you should try and pair a high or medium note with a base note for a longer lasting effect though.

## Make Labels

Again, this need not be anything fancy and is a tool to aid your memory. What can happen if you don't label the jars is that you end up with a cupboard full of half-filled jars of oil that you are too scared to use because you cannot remember what went into them.

Get yourself some of those plain old school book labels and write what oils were used in the blend, and what quantities were used as well. Also make a note of what the blend is meant to do.

Make sure that your hands are clean of any oil residue before writing out the label and wipe down the outside of the bottle for the same reason. Apply the label and immediately cover it with a clear plastic - the self-adhesive type is best.

The reason to protect the label is that, over time, oil will spill out of the jar and if it comes into contact with the label, it can make it illegible.

This little bit of effort won't be a waste of time - simply refill the bottle with the same blend over and over again if it is one that works well.

Cover the label with an adhesive plastic or cello tape so that it is completely protected from cream/ oil spills. (If you don't, the label may become unreadable over time)

If you do get yourself into the situation where you are faced with a blend and you don't know what oils it contains, it is better to throw it out and start again rather than risking using it on your child.

# Patch Tests

I always test any new blend that I make on my inner arm first before I even think of handing it over to someone else. The skin on your inner arm is more sensitive and so if it reacts to the blend, you know immediately that it is too strong for your child to use.

Take a little time to note the way the blend reacts to the skin - does it cause itching and irritation? Does it sting a little? If so, dilute it further and try again. Only once you are absolutely convinced that the oil is non-irritating can you think about using it on your baby's skin.

When you are certain that the blend is good, apply a small amount to your baby's skin to see whether or not there are any bad reactions. Wait at least 12 hours and note if there is any irritation to the skin or any allergic reaction.

If that patch test also comes up clear, you can use the blend on your baby.

Do this for every single oil that you will be applying to your baby's skin. The gentler oils like Lavender and Chamomile are unlikely to stir up an allergic reaction but each child is different - you never know how your baby will react so rather be safe than sorry.

For safety sake, also take this precaution when you are using an older blend that hasn't been used in a while - it is a good way to make sure that the oils haven't become rancid.

When you get a new batch of oils, do the patch test again, just to make sure that there is nothing in the oils that can react with baby's skin. Again, if this is an oil that you have used previously, this is more of a wise precaution than an absolute must but it can pay you to be a bit more careful, especially when it comes to a young baby.

## You Have an Excuse to Keep the Baby Food Jars!

I used to horde these jars - I would carefully wash them out and keep them because I just knew that they would come in handy one day. Baby food jars are ideal for mixing up blends in. All you need to do is to sterilize the bottles first. You can make a nice quantity of mix that will last for a couple of weeks. The bottles have a wide-enough mouth so that you can get to any cream in the bottom of the jar and they are quite easy to use for oils as well.

If you don't have enough baby food jars, just look at your local Dollar Store or Walmart. At a push, check on eBay. Get jars that have a wide mouth and that are shorter so that you can easily get at the contents. I find that jars are easiest overall because you can use them for cream or oils. With bottles, especially those with narrow necks, you have a battle to get an aqueous cream into the bottle and it may be more difficult to get all the cream out again, especially when it comes to a thicker aqueous base.

Glass is a better bet than plastic - it keeps that contents at a more even temperature, is easier to sterilize and easier to keep odor-free once clean. Plastic will do at a push but I wouldn't use it over the long-term as the chemicals in the jar can react to the essentials oils and leach into the oil over time.

There is nothing stopping you from recycling old food jars as well. Just be careful to use jars with close-fitting lids that do not still smell strongly of the food they once contained as this could interfere with your blend - Lavender and vinegar never smell good together.

If you are using a plastic bottle, use it once and then throw it out. If you are using a glass bottle, you can use it several times. It should never be used for food once it has had essential oils in it though.

## Begin With the Lowest Possible Concentration

When it comes to your baby, the weaker the concentration of oils the better it is for your baby. Start off with the lowest possible dose and gauge your baby's reaction. I cannot over-emphasise enough just how powerful essential oils are. One drop is more than enough to add to your baby's blend and you will be surprised how effective even just one drop can be.

If baby shows no sign of improvement, you may then increase the concentration of oils but never exceed the guidelines that I have set out on Chapter 4. This could lead to sensitization or toxicity build-up and neither of these outcomes is what you want for your baby.

When used in the right concentrations, essential oils are a perfectly safe form of therapy. When abused over a longer period of time, they can become dangerous.

I also advise never using an essential oil for longer than 3 weeks of the month in a row. After this, give it a break for about a week before starting up again.

# Chapter 3: The Best Essential Oils to Use for Baby

## These Oils are Your Basic First Aid Kit

Here are the oils that you can choose from as a basic first aid kit for your baby. My top four oils are (in order of importance): Lavender, Chamomile, Eucalyptus and Tea Tree. I do recommend that you buy Lavender and Chamomile to start off with. You may select other oils from the list as you go along.

## From 10 Weeks to 3 Months

### Lavender

Lavender oil has a clean, herbaceous scent and is one of the most versatile oils to have, especially if you have kids. The oil is gentle enough to be used on children from the age of 10 weeks onwards and is wonderfully calming and healing. Most babies do like the smell.

I am pretty sure that this is the oil that you will use most often so I advise that you make up a blend, diluted according to the rules in Chapter 4, to keep ready when necessary.

Many books advise applying Lavender oil neat to skin but I disagree with this. It is okay to do so occasionally when your kids get a little older but, as a general rule, I always dilute the oil before using it. It is just as effective diluted as it is neat and doesn't smell quite as overpowering.

Apply to scratches, minor burns and skin rashes. Rub on sore, hard tummies to relieve an upset tummy or constipation. If your baby is upset or over-tired, Lavender oil can be wonderfully calming. A quick trick to calm baby is to gently massage the lavender blend into the palms of his hands and soles of his feet. This soothes and distracts baby at the same time and can stop a temper tantrum in its tracks.

Lavender diffused in your baby's room will help them to have a peaceful and quiet night's rest - just leave the diffuser on for about half an hour or so and they will calm down. It can help treat allergic reactions and reduce the symptoms of pain and fever.

If there is only one oil that you intend to get, this is it.

Lavender oil, combined with Chamomile oil is one of the most useful, synergistic blends that a parent can have and is likely to be the blend used most often with your baby. This blend is great for using as a nightly massage oil for baby and will help soothe him and boost immunity.

## Chamomile

It is amazing to me how the humble little Chamomile flower can produce such a potent remedy. I still use it in place of Clove oil when I have a toothache and find that it works helps to deaden the pain until I can get to the dentist.

Chamomile is definitely the second-most important essential oil that a parent could have.  It is also gentle enough to be used from ages 10 weeks and up and is a great companion to Lavender oil.

Blend it into an organic aqueous base and you have a soothing, multi-purpose cream that will help fight inflammation and allergic skin conditions. Apply to soothe diaper rash and dry, sensitive skin. Mixing it with Sandalwood or Cedar Wood anchors it and improves the skin soothing action of the oil. (Although these oils should only be introduced when your baby is over 6 months old)

It can also alleviate the pain associated with sunburn and minor burns and help to stimulate the regeneration of damaged skin. Apply in the form of a cold compress as soon as your baby burns themselves and it can help to reduce blistering as well.

Used in a warm compress it can help alleviate pain and fever - it is especially useful when it comes to earache and toothache. Simply soak baby's clean wash cloth in warm water to which you have added a drop of Chamomile oil and a drop of Lavender oil, wring out the cloth and apply to the site of the pain. (On the outside) It is one of the oils with the strongest analgesic properties.

Chamomile can also help you and your spouse get a better night's sleep and feel more relaxed and peaceful.

# Dill

Dill is in the same family as fennel and although they are often interchanged with one another, they are not exactly the same. Dill is milder as an essential oil than Fennel is and does not have as much of diuretic effect.

Dill should be diluted well as it has a detoxifying effect. Use at 0.5% concentration in children up to the age of 2 years old. It is most useful for treating upset tummies but can also be beneficial when it baby has a tight chest or asthma. It is a strong anti-spasmodic.

It blends well with Lavender oil but not with Chamomile oil.

# From 3 Months to 12 Months:

## Tea Tree

This is not one of my favorites but there is no denying that it is effective. It does smell better when mixed with Eucalyptus. It is a potent antibacterial, antiviral and anti-fungal agent.

This is one of those few times when I suggest using an oil neat - when there is a fungal infection like Ringworm, apply the oil neat three to four times a day and continue to apply twice a day for at least another week once the fungal infection has cleared up to prevent reinfection. (But only in children older than a year.)

The oil can be diffused or added to the bath water to chase away the flu virus. Mixed with Eucalyptus oil and a suitable carrier oil, you can use it as a foot rub to help treat colds and the flu and to reduce fevers. Use it in the smallest dilution you can find.

Added to the water used to clean the floors and wipe down the counters, it becomes a valuable natural and anti-bacterial cleaner and will allow you to do away with harsh cleaning chemicals that could be harming the health of your baby.

Using Tea Tree oil, Eucalyptus oil and Lavender oil can in a diffuser will help clear up congestion in baby and prevent the spread of infection.

This is another oil with multiple uses and it has been proven to be as effective as conventional bactericidal agents.

That said, it is not an oil that is easy to blend with others and so you may find that you will use it mainly on its own. For this reason, and because of the strong smell, you may decide to leave this until last when collecting your oils.

# Eucalyptus

Eucalyptus also has quite a strong medicinal smell and is also difficult to blend but I would choose it over Tea Tree oil any day. It has similar anti-viral and antibacterial properties but is also a strong decongestant and can be used very effectively to ease a tight chest or clear up infected sinuses. It does blend well enough with Lavender oil and blends extremely well with Tea Tree oil.

It is also really useful when it comes to treating sore muscles - simply blend with an appropriate carrier oil and massage in or add a few drops to the bath for instant pain relief.

It does help to bring down a fever as well.

Oddly enough, though Tea Tree oil and Eucalyptus oil are difficult to blend when it comes to other oils, they do blend well together to deliver a very strong antibacterial and anti-viral punch and both oils can boost immunity. Mix this blend with Lavender and bacteria and viruses don't stand much of a chance.

# Sandalwood

Sandalwood is one of the world's best loved oils for good reason - it has a reassuring earthy scent and provides a very effective base for blends - it acts as a fixative for the more volatile oils and also contributes a lot to the blend in its own right.

Sandalwood blends with a great many of the other oils and can be used to great effect when it comes to dealing with anxiety. Use with Lavender and Chamomile to soothe baby when he is over-tired or over-anxious.

It is useful in treating dry, sensitive skin and is useful in a blend for treating eczema.

# Neroli

Neroli oil is another of the very calming oils and can be used to help an anxious baby throughout the day. It is one of the easier oils to blend but can be photo-toxic so don't apply it just before going out into the sun.

For the skin, this oil is great as a regenerative treatment - it is good for promoting the healing of wounds that have already closed and for softening scar tissue.

Mixed with Sandalwood and Lavender oil in an appropriate base, it is a really moisturizing treatment for dry and damaged skin and can help baby' skin to regenerate naturally. It should be well-diluted before use.

## Geranium

This has a fairly strong scent and, to me at least, smells more like a herb than a floral scent. It is, however, classified as a floral note and is often used as a replacement for Rose oil in blends.

If baby has eczema or any other kind of skin complaint, you should definitely buy this oils. It is wonderful for treating skin complaints.

It is also calming and helps to relieve anxiety.

It is quite an easy oil to blend but may have the tendency to overpower your blend so it is best to treat it as if it were a base oil.

Blending it with Neroli oil, Palma Rosa Oil and Sandalwood oil makes one of the best skin-soothing blends that you can get for rashes, eczema and other skin complaints.

It is also a great skin re-generator and so is useful in the treatment of scars and burns.

# Bergamot

Bergamot is one of the citrus oils but does not have a distinctly citrus scent. It blends quite well with other oils and is really great for use when it comes to treating troubled, oily skin conditions. Care should be taken as the oil is photo-toxic - it should never be applied just before going out into the sun.

It does have antibacterial properties as well and can be used as an effective remedy for colds and the flu and is also good for treating genito-urinary tract infections. If your baby suffers from thrush, this oil can help.

If insects are pestering your children, add a few drops of Bergamot to the bath water or into a cream base with a few drops of Lavender for an effective insect repellent.

# Rose

Rose is one of those oils that are most likely to be blended with other oils. Be careful to check what it is blended with to ensure that you can use it for your baby.

It blends with just about any other essential oil and lends a deep, exotic fragrance to the blend.

Rose is good for skin ailments - burns, rashes, etc. and has excellent regenerative properties. It pairs especially well with Neroli and Sandalwood oils to help treat dry and sensitive skin.

It helps to calm and soothe baby.

# Palmarosa

This is one of the oils that is derived from a grass. It's most outstanding use is that it is an excellent at promoting skin regeneration and that it can help to balance out all manner of skin complaints. If your baby has any kind of allergic skin reaction, this is one of the oils that you should have on hand.

# Chapter 4: Getting the Dilution Right

## Essential Oils are Very Powerful - Dilute Them for Optimal Results

Here we are going to deal with exactly how the oils should be diluted so that they are safe to use for your baby. In Chapter 3, you learned about some useful oils and about what age groups they were suitable for. It is important to stick to age-appropriate oils. Introducing oils at the wrong age can cause troubles in terms of sensitization and irritation. Some oils are stronger than others and this needs to be kept in mind when it comes to choosing oils for your baby.

I want to stress that dilutions for a baby are far lower than that for an adult because babies are so much smaller. It is always better, when it comes to treating your baby, to err on the side of caution.

The younger the child, the less able they will be to deal with the effects of the oil and the more likely they are to have an adverse reaction. Essential oils can have strong detoxifying properties and not everyone has a system that is strong enough to cope with these effects.

You also need to take the health of your baby into consideration. If they are on the weaker side, half the normal concentration of oils until they start to get stronger again. Otherwise you risk overloading their systems and creating more problems for them.

Don't ever use more oils than is strictly necessary and always follow the guidelines laid out below. Should you wish to increase the concentration of the oils in excess of these guidelines, you must consult a qualified aromatherapist first.

I found that these guidelines were fine for my children. I never felt that I needed to increase the concentrations too much. Essential oils are a lot more powerful than you realize and you need to work within the guidelines to keep your baby safe.

Switching out the oils at least once a month will help to prevent compounds building up in the system and also reduce the chances that a tolerance will develop. Should a tolerance develop, the oils will be much less effective anyway so it is better to give them a break for at least one week out of every month.

## 0-10 Weeks

Remember - essential oils are not to be used until after baby has reached the age of 10 weeks. A baby's skin is a lot more permeable at this age and so more of the oils would be absorbed. Even just one exposure to an essential oil at this stage could cause sensitization to that oil for life. At this age, baby cannot deal with the detoxifying effects of the oils yet.

If your child is sickly or small for his age, wait a little longer before starting with the essential oils treatment. Don't feel impatient at this enforced waiting period - before you know it, the time will have passed and you will be able to treat your baby.

I would also avoid using essential oils on your own person when you are around your baby. This is particularly important if you are breast feeding. Avoid using oils on your breasts anytime near feeding time. Wait at least an hour or two before breast feeding baby to allow the oils to dissipate sufficiently.

# 10 Weeks - 6 Months

At this age, you can start to introduce some of the gentler oils at the lowest concentration.

When using the diffuser, use no more than one or two drops. Expose baby to oils in the diffuser for no more than half an hour a day at most, preferably not in the same room that he spends most of his time in. I suggest using the diffuser outside of the baby's room so that you can limit his exposure - the scent of the oils will be present for a lot longer than half an hour.

When making a blend, the concentration should be 0,5% at most. This translates into 10ml of your chosen base for every drop of essential oil that has been added.

When massaging baby, you must avoid the eyes, nose, mouth and genitals. I advise skipping the face altogether at this stage.

If your baby is congested or has a cold, you can mix 1 drop of Dill oil and 1 drop of Lavender oil in 20ml of a carrier oil and rub it into his feet and his back. If you are finding that this is not sufficient to help clear up the congestion, halve the concentration of the oils and then rub onto your baby's chest.

You may also add the oils of your choice to the baby's bathwater. Never exceed two drops of oil when doing this. The oils will not dissolve in the water so you need to mix them into about 125ml milk before adding them to the water. This helps the oils to disperse more evenly in the water and so reduces the possibility of the oils coming into direct contact with your baby's skin. Alternatively, mix the oils into a bit of honey for a similar effect.

I would probably be described as over-cautious, but once my children got to the age when splashing their bath water all over the place became a very fund game for them, I stopped using the oils in the bath altogether. Personally I find that oils in the bath are more useful for adults treating sore muscles. With babies it is equally easy to add their oils into their daily massage routine.

Oils that you can think about using for your baby at this stage are:

Chamomile, Lavender, Chamomile and Dill.

Eucalyptus, Sweet Orange, Tea Tree oil and Ylang Ylang may be used in a diffuser at this stage in baby's life as they can end up irritating your baby's skin. If you really and truly want to apply these oils in a blend, reduce the concentration to 0.2% and always do a patch test first to make sure that they are diluted enough.

# 6 Months - 2 Years

The concentration of oils stays the same at 0.5% but you no longer have to worry about halving the concentration when rubbing blends into your child's chest.

Babies 6 months and older are a lot better equipped to deal with any side effects that the oils may have. to cope with any effects of the oils.

All of the essential oils listed below can be used at a concentration of 0.5%. (1 drop of essential oil for every 10 ml of carrier oil or base.) and can be used in a diffuser or in a blend.

In addition to Chamomile, Lavender and Dill, you may now also add:

Bergamot, Cedar Wood, Eucalyptus, Frankincense, Ravensara, Sweet Orange, Tea Tree, Ylang Ylang Geranium, Grapefruit, Helichrysum, Neroli, Palmarosa, Rose Otto, Sandalwood.

Essential oils have so many different means of application that if you are worried about causing a reaction in the skin, you can always chose a more indirect application method such as diffusion.

The carrier that you use to blend with the oils helps you to get great effects with only a small amount of oil. You need only drops at a time so they end up being really good value for money.

Try for yourself and see how much even just one drop of oil can scent a carrier. In adults, you will use, at most, a concentration of between 3% and 6% of essential oils to your carrier oil or base.

Try out the different application methods and see which is most convenient for you and for the problem that you are aiming to solve.

Just one note when it comes to choosing carrier oils or creams that you will be using for your baby - choosing an organic cream that is of high quality is really important. The better the quality of your ingredients, the better the action of the blend that you make.

## Inhalation

The easiest way to use essential oils is by diffusing them into the air around you. It is also the safest method when it comes to younger children as there is no contact with the skin. Many oils that are not safe to apply to the skin can because they are irritants can be used in diffusers - all the benefit, none of the irritation. You don't even need to buy a diffuser - there are many different ways to diffuse the oils.

If you need something quick and easy for baby or for a toddler, a bandanna bib is a good alternative. All you have to do is to drop or two of your chosen oils onto the bandanna and then make sure that it is securely tied and that baby cannot get it into his mouth. When fastening the bib, be sure not to make it so tight that baby battles to breathe. You should leave the bib on for a minimum of 20-30 minutes and then give baby a break. The bib can be washed and reused quite easily. This is a really effective way of using essential oils and has the advantage that your whole house does not have to smell of the oils.

What I used to do with my kids was to knit them a cuddle buddy - there are patterns all over the Internet - I would then cut a patch of matching fabric into the shape of a heart and applique it on, leaving one side open. I then took a plain piece of cotton and added a drop of Lavender oil and a drop of Chamomile oil to it and then placed this cotton inside the patch before hand-stitching it closed. The scent permeated the fabric heart and the heart prevented my kids from coming into direct contact with the oils. This helped keep them calm and helped them to sleep at night. We still have a couple of cuddly buddies out in the garage - my kids will not let me throw them out.

An aromatherapy burner is a relatively inexpensive piece of equipment and very easy to get. You do need to take care though that the whole setup is kept out of the child's reach. Many people have switched over to electronic diffusers in place of burners because they are safer to use and because there is some fear that the actual heating or essential oils may alter the compounds within leaving them less effective.

I never had an electronic diffuser when my kids were little and so I used an aromatherapy burner. I don't feel that the efficacy of the oils is damaged by heating them up so I have no problems with using a burner.

I use a diffuser today though because it is a lot simpler and a lot safer than using a candle.

If you have a radiator, you can also set a bowl of water near enough so that the water can evaporate. Add in a couple of drops of the essential oils of your choice but do make sure that your kids are unable to reach the bowl.

## Bath Water and Showering

As mentioned above, the oils do not actually disperse in the water but rather sit on the surface. The water temperature helps the oils to evaporate so that the benefit of the scent is obtained. The oils will also be absorbed into the skin.

There is a possibility, when using oils in the bath, that the oils may irritate your child's skin. It is for this reason that it is advisable to mix the oils with glycerin, a little bit of honey or some milk before adding them to the bath. Milk can be wonderfully soothing for dry, sensitive skin so add up to half a cup to your child's bath water as necessary.

I was always worried that the milk would leave a sour smell on the skin afterwards - I guess I thought it would go off but it is all absorbed by the skin and is a a really soothing treatment - just as good for moms and dads as it it for kiddies.

Add 1-2 drops of oil to half a cup of milk or a tablespoon of honey/glycerin and add to bath water just before you put your kids into bath.

If your kids are a little older and use the shower rather than the bath, dampen a wash cloth, add a couple of drops of essential oils and put it on the floor of the shower just before they climb in. The heat in the shower will help the oils to evaporate and the scent will permeate the air.

# Oils in a Cream Base

Aqueous cream is a staple in our home. It is great to use as a carrier for oils and provides a non-greasy alternative to carrier oils. If you want a base that is lighter than an oil, an aqueous cream is a really good alternative. Look for a cream that is organic and that has no scent or coloring. If possible, find a herbal center in the area and get them to make up the aqueous base for you.

When it comes to petroleum-based creams, I suggest only using these when it is absolutely necessary. I find that these creams are often less nourishing and substantial than those based on plant-oils.

I really feel that it is worthwhile to use a good, organic, plant-based aqueous cream because of the benefits for your skin. I have used petroleum-based products in an effort to save a bit of money but have always gone back to the organic base. The organic cream seems to be a lot more effective and really sinks into the skin. With the petroleum-based products I find that I have to use more cream to get the same effect so it works out at about the same cost-wise anyway.

If your child has a skin problem such as eczema, it is even more important to source a great naturally based product. Sweet almond oil is useful for soothing troubled skin and so is Helichrysum. You can add up to 10% - 20% of carrier oils to the aqueous cream base and still retain the creamy texture.

Follow the rules for Chapter 3, according to the age of your child. If possible, use a glass jar to store the cream in. I always used to wash out the baby food jars very well before standing them in boiling water to sterilize them. I find that they are a nice size to make up just enough cream for about a week or so and they are easy to store.

Add the cream to the jar, and then add your oils. Start with the lowest concentration first and do the smell test after each oil is added. If you accidentally add too much by way of essential oils, simply increase the amount of aqueous cream accordingly. Once you are satisfied with your blend, mix it up and seal. I find that a wooden skewer is easiest because of the size of the bottle but you can also use the back of a dinner spoon. I prefer the skewers because you can just throw them out after using them.

I let the cream sit overnight before using it so that the oils really have time to permeate the cream.

Always, when using the blend for the first time, do a patch test on your child's skin first and wait at least 6 hours to ensure that there is no adverse reaction to the blend.

## Carrier Oils

There is a lot to be said for carrier oils. I used to balk at the idea of using an oil on my kids, thinking it would be too greasy. The key is to choose the right carrier oil and to get a good quality oil. Cheaper oils are less refined and are not as easily absorbed. They are also more likely to be blended with cheaper and more common oils like sunflower oil so do do a little research before buying your oil. I do find that oil blends are more useful in the winter months as well, when the skin is more likely to be chapped and dry and in need of a little more care.

You can also choose the type of carrier oil to help treat your child's condition. Oils like Sweet Almond oil and Grape Seed oil are suitable for use on all skin types and are good oils to keep at the ready for general conditions. I feel it is worthwhile getting a slightly bigger bottle of these generally useful carrier oils because you will use them so often. I find that a 500ml - 1 liter bottle is best as it saves me running to the store too often to replace it.

Unless your child has eczema, steer clear of the heavier oils such as avocado or macadamia and, when using them, dilute them with a lighter oil - they should be a maximum of 50% concentration or the blend will not be as easily absorbed and will not feel nice on the skin. They are simply too rich to be used as they are. When buying oils that are high in monounsaturated fats, like Avocado and Macadamia, get a smaller bottle as a little goes such a long way that you will not use them up very quickly. In many cases you can get away with a concentration of only 10% of these oils in a carrier oil.

Extra-virgin Olive oil can make a good stand-in for the other oils. It makes a nice change from Sweet Almond and Grape Seed and has antibacterial properties as well. It is also quite rich. Just be sure that you get pure Olive Oil as the cheaper brands tend to be diluted with other seed oils that are not as nice on the skin. The extra virgin Olive Oil has a much nicer texture than plain old Olive oil that you cook with and is absorbed much more easily.

You can also use sunflower oil at a stretch but really only for massage oils. I advise against using sunflower oil on the face. It is a lot heavier than the other oils and is not as easily absorbed. If using sunflower oil, I recommend rubbing it in and leaving it on for about 10-15 minutes. Then go back and remove any excess oils.

Bathing or showering can help to increase the absorption of the oil and wash away the unnecessary excess.

## Sweet Almond Oil and Apricot Kernel Oil

These oils come from the same broad family and have very similar qualities. They are both nutrient-rich oils and suitable for dry or troubled skin. They are pretty much inter-changeable but Sweet Almond oil is usually more affordable.

Both oils can help to promote cell regeneration and healing and are great to use to reduce scarring. If your child has eczema, these oils can prove extremely useful in helping to provide relief from the itching and dryness. If your child has an allergy to nuts, you should take care when using this oil.

Sweet Almond oil is alright to use when treating acne if the underlying skin is dry and sensitive. If the skin is more oily, Grape Seed oil is the better choice.

## Avocado Oil

Avocado oil is too rich to be used on its own so always dilute it in equal parts with another oil when treating a really bad skin condition or use it in a concentration of 10% on skin that just needs a bit of a healing boost. This oil is good for treating eczema and can help to heals burns, scars and sunburn. It is best to buy only a little at a time - a little of the oil goes a long way but the oil itself can turn rancid more rapidly than other oils.

## Helichrysum Oil

This is one of the big heroes when it comes to troubled skin - it is great for moisturizing dry or dehydrate skin, treating rashes, bruises and eczema and can help to heal acne and prevent scarring. Use in a 10% concentration for best results.

Add about a tablespoon of the oil to your baby's bum cream once they are over 10 weeks old and see and you will not battle as much with chafing or rashes.

It can be a helpful treatment for teething pains - simply mix with equal quantities of Sweet Almond/ Grape Seed oil and add in

Lavender and Chamomile oil in the correct dilutions and apply to the outside of the jaw and just under the cheekbones.

It is also a useful oil to use when your child has Chicken Pox and can reduce the itchiness and the chances that the pustules will burst and leave scars.

## Coconut Oil

Coconut oil is best avoided when it comes to small children as it can cause rashes. If you really want to try it, use it on a small area at first and watch carefully to see if any rashes develop. I would still reserve it for use on children older than 6 to avoid possible sensitization later on. The oil itself has strong anti-bacterial and anti-fungal properties but you can get the benefits of these by using it as a cooking oil as well.

It is a very moisturizing oil and does make a good base for lip balms and body butters as it is semi-solid at room temperature.

## Grape Seed Oil

Sweet Almond and Grape Seed oils are popular because they are non-sensitizing and stable. Grape Seed oil is not as nourishing as Sweet Almond oil and has a slightly astringent quality but is better for skins that are on the oilier side.

## Jojoba Oil/ Wax

This is actually solid at normal room temperature and so makes a good base for lip balms and body butters - you'll never run out of gifts for teachers or your child's friends. It is non-comdagenic, which means that it does not block up the pores. It is a good addition to acne creams and can be useful in soothing inflamed skin. It has good staying power because it does not oxidize as easily as some other oils and it is often used as a base oil to stabilize other more volatile oils.

## Macadamia Nut

Macadamia Nut oil is very nutritious and good for treating dry or sun-burnt skin. I would only use it on kids older than 6 years old to prevent possible allergies developing. It makes a good addition to a day cream - use it in a 10% - 15% concentration to help soothe skin and to help protect against damage from the sun.

## Wheatgerm Oil

Again, keep this oil for kids over the age of 6 to avoid possible allergies developing. It is a particularly healing oil when it comes to acne in that it moisturizes the skin and helps it to heal. It is also really good for an allergic rash or eczema and helpful in treating muscles that are sore and stiff.

Always dilute it with another oil. It should compose no more than 10% of your blend.

# Special Treatment Oils

These should only be used in cases where the condition warrants it and never on children under the age of 6 months old, to avoid possible allergies developing. Keep the dilution to maximum of 10% of the blend and mix in well with the other carrier oil. Before using the blend be sure to shake well again in case the oils have separated.

When my kids were small, I really only used Avocado oil as a treatment oil. The oils that I have listed below can be helpful but I would really only get them if you would be able to use them as well.

At the small concentrations we are talking about, this can end up being an expensive purchase otherwise.

## Borage Oil

This is not always that easy to find but makes a great addition to a blend for irritated skin. It calms irritation and provides essential fatty acids that the skin needs. It is also a good oil to use when skin is damaged or scarred. Use diluted with a carrier oil at about 10% strength. Evening Primrose oil is a good substitute for Borage oil and has very similar properties.

## Carrot Oil

Helps to calm and heal irritated skin. It promotes regeneration of the skin and is useful in the treatment of acne. Again, use at about 10% concentration.

## Castor Oil

You'll probably know this more as a laxative than anything else. It is not a pleasant oil to apply to the skin because it has a sticky texture. It can be helpful in bringing a boil to a head or in healing sores and abscesses. If your child is suffering from constipation, you can mix this with another oils at about 10% concentration and rub into the abdominal area.

## Cocoa Butter

This is extremely nourishing and is especially useful for dry skin.

## Linseed Oil

This is an oil that is very good for skin that is irritated. Apply as a spot treatment for acne to reduce redness and swelling.

## Meadow Sweet Oil

Helps to fight pain and inflammation. It is quite a good oil for muscle soreness.

## Peanut Oil

This has strong analgesic properties. I would not use it on a child under the age of 6 for fear of allergies developing. Rub into sprains and sore muscles for relief.

## Rosehip Oil

This has the highest concentration of Vitamin C and helps to heal and regenerate skin. It helps to treat scarring and is a very effective moisturizer. Added to a night cream blend, at about 10% concentration, this is a winning remedy for treating acne.

## St John's Wort/ Hypericum

This can be blended in equal parts with Helychrisum oil to create a really healing treatment for burned skin and to reduce scarring overall.

# Chapter 5: Daily Massage for Your Baby

## Using the Power of Touch to Make Your Baby Happy

Massaging your baby has a lot of positive effects for both of you.

This is not a massage in the sense that you are working to release knots and tension, it is more a series of fluid motions and gentle tugs. Massage can help the two of you to bond and help to keep your baby's nervous system healthy. It relaxes baby's body, keeps the limbs limber and helps to encourage the circulation. This is very beneficial to baby and helps to improve his physical and mental health and boosts immunity.

Small children need physical touch to reassure them that they are loved and cared for - a daily massage will help baby feel more reassured and loved.

You should should skip the massage if your baby is sick, has just been immunized, or if they have a full tummy. Also never massage just before a feeding. If the skin is broken or newly scarred, avoid the area completely until it has healed.

Make sure that you work on a comfortable surface - baby's changing mat is ideal and make sure that the room temperature is warm - your baby is not as easily able to deal with cold as you are.

Once baby is over 10 weeks old, the following blend makes a very soothing massage oil:

1 drop Lavender oil

1 drop Chamomile oil

20ml Sweet Almond oil

The Lavender and Chamomile oils both help to boost immunity and calm baby. The blend will help to keep baby's skin healthy and will aid digestion as well. The blend is gentle enough to be used every day.

When doing the massage for the first time, rub some of the blend between your palms and move closer to your baby. What does he seem to think of the smell? If he has no reaction, that is fine. If he starts to cry and pull away, you will need to think of something else as he does not like the blend.

If that is okay, do a small patch test and wait for at least 12 hours to see whether or not there is a bad reaction to the blend.

If all is good after this, warm a little of the oil by rubbing it between the palms of your hands and begin the massage. Start at your baby's feet and gently rub the oils in. You can gently push up against baby's feet so that his leg muscles are strengthened. My kids used to think that this was great fun and an opportunity to kick me. Don't worry about this, he will settle down as the massage proceeds.

A quick little game of "This Little Piggy" can help to start the massage off on the right foot by relaxing baby.

Move up the leg and GENTLY tug at it - this is just to stretch the legs out a little so don't pull too had.

Move up to the thighs using a gentle, rhythmic movement. Avoid the genital area and proceed to the tummy. Gently rub the tummy using circular movements before moving onto the chest. Again, use circular motions. Then move onto the the hands and repeat the motions that you used with the feet, this time playing "Pat a Cake" rather than "This Little Piggy".

If baby allows you to, roll him over onto his tummy and massage his back by running one hand down the spine before repeating with the other hand.

Finish off by giving baby a big cuddle before dressing him again. Talk to baby throughout - even if it is only to tell him what it is that you are doing.

Done every evening, this will help baby relax and sleep a whole lot better.

# Chapter 6: Essential Oils for the Skin

## Dealing with Common Skin Issues That Babies May Have

Many babies have sensitive skin and are prone to common skin complaints like eczema. They will often grow out of it but while they are battling with these skin complaints, they can be very uncomfortable. Luckily, essential oils can be used from a very early age to help relieve the symptoms.

If your child has sensitive skin it is very important that any blend that you make up is tested on a small patch of skin before you lather it on the whole body. Using the wrong oil can result in sensitive skin flaring up very badly so it is well worth taking this extra precaution here.

You will also have to look beyond what oils you can apply to the skin after bathing but also to all the products that you use on your baby's skin. Normal soap is far too harsh so find an appropriate baby shampoo. If need be, you can use this as a cleanser on the skin as well.

Being more careful about bath time procedures is also a good idea - when you take your baby out of the bath, cuddle him on a nice, soft towel and dab the skin dry. Applying too much pressure by rubbing your child's skin dry can lead to outbreaks. While still in the bathroom, apply your chosen blend - cream is normally better for skin conditions as oils can be too heavy and overload the skin.

Apply the blend every morning and evening for best results and repeat throughout the day if you find it necessary to do so.

It also pays to dress your baby in natural fibers as far as possible as these allow the skin to breathe. Synthetic fibers can promote overheating of the skin and this can make problem areas even worse.

Here are some oils commonly used for skin ailments, just check in chapter 4 for the right concentrations to use for general conditions and you can use this as a guide when making up your own blends. If you are not keen to make your own blends yet, I have included some recipes at the end of this chapter.

**Antiseptics for cuts, insect bites, infected rashes, etc:** Making baby understand that he should not scratch itchy spots and rashes is not possible so you need to have some form of antiseptic oil on hand should the spot get infected. For babies between the ages of 10 weeks and 6 months, use Lavender oil. For those up to the age of 2 years, use Eucalyptus oil and Tea Tree oil, for older children use Thyme oil, Clary Sage oil, and Lemon oil. All of the oils should be diluted well before application. Apply at least two to three times a day.

**Anti-inflammatory oils for eczema, infected wounds, bumps, bruises, etc:** For babies ages of 10 weeks and up, use Chamomile oil , Lavender oil and Yarrow oil. Whether you use an oil or a lotion will depend on the condition being treated - for bruises, either is fine; for eczema, the treatment will be based on whether the eczema is dry or weeping - weeping eczema responds better to a light cream, dry eczema responds better to an oils based treatment. Apply at least twice daily for optimal results.

**Fungicidal oils for Candida, ringworm, etc:** For babies between the ages of 10 weeks and 6 months, use Lavender oil and apply neat. For babies over the ages of 6 months, you can use Tea Tree oil neat and Myrrh oil, Patchouli oil and Sweet Marjoram oil in a well-diluted format. Choose the best base for your baby. Olive oil has a strong anti-fungal action so it would make a good base. Apply 4-5 times daily and, once the site has cleared, continue to apply twice daily for at least 7 days to make sure that the fungal infection is well and truly dead.

**Healing oils for burns, cuts, scars, etc:** For children between the ages of 10 weeks and 6 months, use Lavender oil and Chamomile oil. For ages 6 months and up use, Rose, Neroli, Frankincense and Geranium. If there is really bad scarring, you can add in Rose Hip oil to strength of about 5% to the the blend in order to promote healing, as long as baby is older than 6 months. Oils that have a higher proportion of fatty acids in them, such as Macadamia nut and Avocado oil can also be added to the blend .

The following recipes are for creams that can assist in the treatment of eczema and dry, flaky skin:

# Basic Blend for Skin that is Dry and Flaky

(Safe for ages 10 weeks and up)

1 Drop Chamomile oil

1 Drop Lavender oil

Mix into 30ml of a rich, organic aqueous cream. Add in 5ml of Helychrisum oil or Avocado oil and mix well. Apply to affected areas at least twice daily.

## Blend for Eczema, Chapped Skin and Diaper Rash

(Safe from the age of 6 months)

I am going to bet that you will use this blend quite a bit - it is really soothing for the skin at all ages. I use it for my whole family when they have rough dry skin, chapped skin or when they have a rash or itchy bite. I also keep some in the kitchen for when I burn my fingers on the stove - I do that a lot - or when I am working with my hot glue gun. It is very soothing for those minor burns and quickly takes the sting out of the burn.

I use this blend on my face as well - I rate it as the best blend for treating most skin conditions because it helps the skin regenerate and helps moisturize it. (Think I sound a bit like a snake oil salesman? Try the blend, you will love it as much as I do.)

5 drops of Geranium oil

5 drops of Palm Rosa oil

10 drops of Lavender oil

5 drops of Sandalwood oil

250ml organic aqueous cream

Mix all the ingredients well and apply as needed.

## Heat Rash Blend

(Suitable for ages 10 weeks and up)

2 drops Rose oil

2 drops Chamomile oil

2 drops Lavender oil

50ml Rose Water or Rose Hydrosol

Mix all ingredients and shake well. Dab directly onto the rash for instant relief from itching.

Alternatively, add the mixture to a bowl of cool water, soak a wash cloth in it and then wring it out and use the cloth as a cold compress to help reduce itching and swelling.

Alternatively, half the ingredients and add them to 125ml milk to add to baby's bath water.

## Psoriasis Cream

(For ages 6 months and up)

5 drops Lavender oil

5 drops Myrrh

5 drops Tea Tree oil

10ml Avocado oil

10ml Borage oil

200ml thick Aqueous cream

Blend together and apply as needed.

Another option is to replace the Borage oil and aqueous cream with a cup of Apple Cider Vinegar to use as a direct treatment for the spots or use just a drop of each oil and the apple cider vinegar and add to baby's bath water.

## Cold Compresses for Relieving Eczema

If the skin is hot and inflamed, a cold compress can quickly bring relief. For children between the ages of 10 weeks and 6 months, use Lavender oil and Chamomile oil - put one drop of each oil into your bowl of water before soaking a wash cloth in it. Wring out and apply to the affected area. Soak a second wash cloth and use alternately until the discomfort has been eased.

If the child is older than 6 months, add 2 drops of either Lavender or Chamomile and 2 drops of any ONE of the following oils:

**To treat weepy eczema:** Myrrh or Patchouli

**To treat scaly eczema:** Melissa or Rose

**To treat inflamed eczema:** Chamomile or Yarrow

**To treat infected eczema:** Tea Tree or Lavender.

# For Insect Bites, Burns and Stings

It is inevitable that your child will be bitten or stung by some insect or another at some stage or another. In the case of a sting, take a credit card and scrape over the area to remove the stinger (pulling it out will only result in more toxins entering the system). If it is the first time your child has been stung, I advise heading to the emergency room as a precautionary measure, in case they are allergic.

You can treat minor burns at home but for anything more serious, head to the emergency room. For a minor burn, apply a cold compress with 2 drops Lavender oil and 2 drops Chamomile or Geranium oils.

Bites and stings can be itchy and/ or painful and inflamed so, once you have established that your child will not have an allergic reaction, you need to apply oils that have calming properties. Here are some recipes to try:

## Compress for Bee Stings/ Itchy Bites

(Suitable for all ages)

This blend is also extremely useful when it comes to treating sunburn.

5ml Baking Soda

2 drops Lavender oil

2 Drops Chamomile oil

Mix the baking soda in a little water until it forms a paste and then mix that into a bowl of icy water. Add in the oils and then soak a clean wash cloth in the mixture for a couple of minutes. Apply to the area for instant relief.

## Soothing Bath for Sunburn

(Suitable for all ages)

2 drops Lavender oil

2 drops Chamomile oil

100ml milk

50ml Baking Soda

Draw a tepid bath and add the baking soda while the water is being poured to help it to dissolve properly. Mix the oils in the milk and add to the water just before your child gets in. Allow them to soak for at least 15-20 minutes.

# Chapter 7: Essential Oils for the Digestive System

## From an Sore Tummy to Diarrhea, Oils Can Be Most Helpful

Your baby will not be able to tell you outright that his tummy is sore but you will be able to tell if this is the case if his tummy is hard and bloated. You will also notice a change in his poop, or lack thereof.

If your baby is between 10 weeks and 6 months old, soak a wash cloth in a bowl of warm water. (This is not a compress, though you can make one up if you prefer to.) Mix 1 drop of Chamomile oil and 1 drop of Lavender oil with 20ml of the carrier oil of your choice or aqueous cream and gently massage it into his abdomen, using one big circular movement and massaging clock-wise. When you are finished, wring out the wash cloth quickly and place it over his tummy. Leave in place for about 5 minutes.

The heat from the cloth has a dual purpose - it helps to relieve the pain of the sore tummy and it helps the oils to be absorbed better. You can replace the Chamomile oil with dill oil in need.

## Blend for a Sore Tummy

(Suitable for ages 10 weeks and up)

1 drop Lavender oil

1 drop Dill oil

20ml carrier oil of your choice

Mix all the ingredients and gently rub into tummy area and abdomen. To aid absorption and give further comfort, apply a warm wash cloth after applying the oils.

# Blend for Colic

(Suitable for ages 10 weeks and up)

1 drop Mandarin oil or 1 drop Sweet Orange oil

1 drop of Lavender oil

20ml of the carrier oil that you prefer.

Mix all the ingredients together and massage the mixture into into the back, chest and abdomen twice daily until the symptoms subside.

# Blend for Diarrhea

(Suitable for ages 6 months and up)

1 drop Lavender oil

1 drop Ginger oil

1 drop Geranium oil

30ml carrier oil of your choice

Mix up all the oils and massage gently into the whole abdomen, again using circular movements. Put a warm wash cloth onto the abdomen afterwards to help speed absorption and help reduce cramping and discomfort.

If your baby has diarrhea, it is important that he gets in enough fluids, even if he will not eat. If this mixture does not stop the diarrhea in a day or if the baby also has a high fever, get him to the emergency room as soon as possible.

## Tummy Rub for Babies Prone to Upsets

(Suitable for ages 10 weeks and up)

1 drop Lavender oil

1 drop Tea Tree oil

20 ml carrier oil of your choice

Massage into baby's belly every alternate morning instead of using the Lavender/ Chamomile combo in order to help kill off gastric bugs before they strike.

# Chapter 8: Essential Oils for Teething

## Help Baby Through this Painful Stage of Development

Teething is a trying time for any baby. They don't really understand what is going on, their mouths may be sore and they may have itchy gums. Help your baby deal with the difficult developmental stage by using essential oils. Chamomile is a particularly good choice because it has strong pain-relieving properties and can help to soothe a frustrated baby.

## Blend to Help Reduce Teething Pain

(Suitable for ages 10 weeks and up)

1 drop Lavender oil

1 drop Chamomile oil

20ml carrier oil of your choice

Apply to the face along the jawline, just under the cheekbones and to the neck and chin to help alleviate tooth ache and teething pain. Reapply two to three times a day. This remedy is extremely effective and has the added benefit of being very calming for the child as well.

# Compress to Relieve Teething Pain

(Suitable for ages 10 weeks and up)

1 drop Chamomile oil

1 drop Lavender oil

1 bowl warm water

Mix all the ingredients together and soak a clean wash cloth in the mixture for a few minutes. Hold the cloth against the jaw where the teeth are coming in to help reduce the pain overall.

# Relief Blend for Bad Teething Pain

(Suitable for ages 6 months and up)

I just want to preface this by saying that I don't like using Clove oil where kids are concerned. It is a very good remedy and a strong antiseptic but I feel that it can be a bit too harsh for baby's skin. However, if your baby is really struggling badly with teething pain, a well-diluted blend of Clove Bud oil can really be useful. Use this mix if your baby is battling with teething but make sure it does not get into his mouth and just watch for out for irritation of the skin. If the skin becomes irritated, I advise either lowering the concentration of Clove Bud oil or swapping it out for Chamomile oil, for a couple of days at least.

1 drop Clove Bud oil

2 drops Lavender oil

50ml carrier oil of your choice

Blend all the oils together and rub only on the areas were the teeth are starting to come in. Be especially careful not to apply this oil too near to the nose or eyes as it can irritate the mucous membranes and can cause eyes to tear up and noses to run.

If that does happen, wipe the oils off baby's face and apply some aqueous cream. You might want to also add a little milk to the water to help soothe the skin more.

# Chapter 9: Essential Oils for Infectious Illness and Fever

## Dealing With Childhood Illnesses That Might Crop Up

For a baby, the most dangerous part of any illness is the fever that develops. If you can manage to break the fever, you can reduce the risk of permanent damage being done.

There are plenty of essential oils that can help you to beat a fever but I do advise some caution here. If your baby is running a very high fever and you are not able to bring it down with a cool compress, it is better to get him to the doctor or emergency room as quickly as possible.

The fever is a sign that your child is fighting an infection, the higher the fever, the worse the infection is and the greater the chances of permanent damage being done to your child. If the fever gets too high, it may cause seizure or it could even be fatal so don't mess around. If the fever is 103 F, it is considered high and you should get proper medical assistance.

If you are treating your child at home, do ensure that he is getting enough liquids. It is best to dilute sugary drinks like fruit juices quite well before giving them to him.

## Reducing Fever With Essential Oils

Cool compresses and tepid baths are your best tools when it comes to beating a high fever. You should never use an ice cold bath as this can be too much for your baby's system to take. A cool compress applied to the back of the neck and to the forehead can help a lot. You can also rinse baby's wrists in cool water to help reduce his fever.

I also found that applying a cool compress under baby's armpits helped quite a bit when he had a stubborn fever. It may have looked a little strange but it was helpful.

For a slightly raised temperature, a cool compress placed on the forehead or behind the neck can be very useful. Alternatively, bathe the child in water that is tepid - cold water can be too much of a shock to the system.

The following oils  are cooling and will help to bring down a fever - make a blend of oil to rub in - rubbing the oils into the back of the neck and feet is best, add to the bath water or use in a cold compress:

For children between the ages of 10 weeks and 6 months use Lavender oil and Chamomile oil.

For children 6 months and older, use the following oils at the normal dilutions: Bergamot oil, Eucalyptus oil, Ginger oil, Helichrysum oil, Lemon oil, Lime oil, Niaouli oil, Rosewood oil, Tea Tree oil, Yarrow oil.

These oils can be used at half the normal dilution:  Basil oil, Juniper oil, Lemongrass oil, Peppermint oil & Spearmint oil, Myrtle oil, Rosemary oil, Sage oil, Thyme oil and Yarrow oil.

# I've Got a Fever Bath

(Suitable for ages 6 months and up)

1 drop Peppermint oil

1 drop Tea Tree oil

1 drop Eucalyptus oil

Draw a bath that feels lukewarm - not hot and cold and add the oils to the water just before you put your baby into it. Sponge the water over the child - from head to foot, avoiding the face. You can sponge the water over the back of the head, just make sure the the water will not drip into baby's face.

You can use a large bowl of water in place of a bath if you have no access to a bath. The procedure is the same except that you would use halve the above-mentioned quantities of oils.

## Fever Foot Rub

(Suitable for ages 6 months and up)

This blend is very effective for drawing down a fever. Be sure to apply it last thing at night and your baby will not only sleep better but will also wake up feeling a lot better as well.

2 drops Eucalyptus oil

2 drops Lemon oil

2 drops Tea Tree oil

60ml carrier oil of your choice

Mix everything together well and then rub into the sole of each foot gently. In need, also rub a small amount of the oil into the back of the neck and chest, if baby is congested. Apply morning, noon and evening for best results. The feet are a particularly good place to apply oils - they are absorbed very quickly into the feet.

# Treating Infectious Illnesses

**Chickenpox:** For children between the ages of 10 weeks and 6 months, use Lavender oil and Chamomile oil. For children 6 months and over, use: Bergamot oil, Eucalyptus oil, and Tea Tree oil. A blend made up of equal parts Lavender oil, Eucalyptus oil and Tea Tree oil, appropriately diluted will help infected spots to heal. An appropriately diluted mix of equal parts of Chamomile oil and Lavender oil will soothe itching and help to prevent scarring, inflammation and infections.  Bathe your baby every 2-3 hours in a tepid bath to which you have added a handful of colloidal oatmeal, 2 drops of Lavender oil, two drops of Tea Tree oil and a teaspoon of Witch Hazel. Alternatively, for children older than 2 years, mix 50ml Rose Water and 50ml Witch Hazel with 5 drops Tea Tree oil, 5 Drops Lavender oil and 5 drops Chamomile oil and dab onto spots.

**Measles:** For children between the ages of 10 weeks and 6 months, use Lavender oil and Chamomile oil. For children 6 months and older, use Bergamot oil, Eucalyptus oil,and Tea Tree oil. If your baby is running a mild temperature, draw a bath as hot as baby can comfortably manage  and add a few drops of Lavender oil and Chamomile oil. Allow them to soak for at least 15 minutes to reduce aching. The steam will be beneficial in opening up airways if this is a concern. If your baby is running a higher temperature is on the higher side, draw a tepid bath to which you add 2 drops of Lavender oil and 1 drop of Tea Tree oil.

# Detoxing the System

These oils  can help to encourage the child to sweating out the toxins and may be added to the bath  water or mixed into a blend - Be sure to choose oils that are  appropriate for your baby's age - this treatment is not suitable to be used in babies under the age of 12 months old and in children that have been diagnosed as having epilepsy: Rosemary, Thyme, Hyssop, Chamomile.

If your child is a blocked nose or tight chest, has a bad cough, sinusitis or bronchitis, and is older than 6 months old, use: Eucalyptus, Pine, Thyme, Myrrh, Sandalwood, Fennel. If your child is between 10 weeks and 6 months old, use Dill oil.

The following oils can be assist in getting rid of dry coughs and whooping cough: Hyssop, Cedar Wood, Bergamot, Chamomile. Only Chamomile is suitable for children between the ages of 10 weeks and  6 months old.

Resinous oils can help in treating the symptoms of colds and congestion and can ward off the chills: Benzoin, Frankincense, Balsam, Myrrh. These oils are only suitable for use in babies  older than 6 months.

The following oils can assist in the treatment of most of the symptoms of colds and the flu: Balsam, Basil, Bergamot, Cinnamon leaf, Citronella, Clove Bud, Coriander, Eucalyptus, Frankincense, Ginger, Grapefruit, Helichrysum, Juniper, Lemon, Lime, Sweet Marjoram, Peppermint & Spearmint, Myrtle, Niaouli, Sweet Orange, Pine, Rosemary, Rosewood,   Clary Sage, Tea Tree, Thyme, Yarrow. Yarrow is the only oil that can be used on a baby that is between 10 weeks and 6 months old. All the other oils should be diluted well.

# Cold and Flu Remedy

(Suitable for ages 10 weeks and up)

1 drop Tea Tree oil

1 drop Eucalyptus oil

For children that are 6 months old or older, you can add these oils to 20ml of carrier oil and rub them into the feet, back and chest. This blend can help with the aches and pains associated with colds and the flu and may, alternatively be added into about 125ml of milk for use in the bath water. For babies under 6 months old, you should only use these oils in a diffuser and at very weak concentrations. Eucalyptus will help unblock a congested nose in a few minutes so keep these sessions with the diffuser confined to 20 minutes at most for smaller babies.

# Infection Killing Bath

(Suitable for children 6 months and older only)

2 drops Eucalyptus oil

2 drops Juniper Berry oil

2 drops Sweet Orange oil

125ml milk

Mix all the oils and milk together and draw a warm bath. Add the oils and allow the baby to soak for about 15 minutes. The heat from the bath will help the oils to evaporate and help to clear up congestion. The oils themselves are good anti-viral and antibacterial agents and will also help to reduce pain and fever.

Alternatively, swap out the milk for 60ml of a carrier of your choice and rub into baby's back, neck and feet. This recipe is only suitable for children aged 12 and older as it is detoxifying and raises the blood pressure. It is not suitable for use if the child has epilepsy.

## Cold and Flu Beating Remedy

(Suitable for ages 6 and up)

60ml carrier oil of your choice

2 drops eucalyptus

2 drops tea tree oil

2 drops mandarin oil

Blend the oils together and ensure that they are well combined. Use as a massage oil, concentrating on the back and the feet. This oil should be applied last thing at night to baby's feet and neck to help clear congestion and enable him to have a good night's sleep.

You can also omit the carrier oil and use the oils in a diffuser or halve the oils and add to 125 ml milk in place of a carrier oil if you want to add them to baby's bath water.

## Cold and Flu Diffuser Blend

(Suitable for ages 6 months and up)

2 drops Tea Tree oil

2 drops Eucalyptus oil

2 drops Lavender oil

This blend will help to clear away the germs in the air and also help to clear up any congestion baby has.

You can, alternatively, add 60ml of a carrier oil of your choice to the blend and use as a massage oil for baby.

# Chapter 10: Essential Oils to Improve Immunity

## Boosting Your Baby's Immune System for Optimal Health

I can be quite mercurial at times - I love sunny days but I also love cold weather. Admittedly though, the cold is not always that great when you have a small baby, especially if they attend daycare. It often takes just one kid to pick up a bug and then they all get it. Without fail, my kids would get at least one cold of bout of flu every year.

And there is not all that much that your doctor can do for them - they can help manage the symptoms and after that your child will simply have to ride it out. Nowadays we understand that antibiotics are pretty much useless against viruses and we also know that most colds and flu are caused by viruses.

To make matters worse is the advent of the super-bugs - drug resistant strains of illnesses that have become immune to the standard antibiotics, precisely because they have been over-used. Antibiotics should be a last resort when it comes to your baby - they wipe out a lot of beneficial bugs as well and can take a toll on your baby's system as well.

In fact, the more synthetic chemicals that you can avoid putting into your baby's system the better. Your baby needs to be exposed to some germs and actually needs to get sick in order to build up their immune systems. It has been proven, contrary to what you might believe, that children that grew up with pets in the health actually develop stronger immune systems and tend to suffer less when it comes to allergies.

Essential oils can be used effectively to help build up your baby's immunity. While I cannot say that my children never got sick, they certainly didn't pick up every single little bug going around and they tended to have less severe symptoms and bounce back faster when they were ill.

I credit that to essential oils and science is now bearing me out. Tea Tree oil and Eucalyptus oil, for example, are very potent immune boosters. They also kill germs very effectively and can slow down viruses as well.

These are just two of the better known oils - all essential oils have antibacterial capabilities and a lot of them are effective antivirals as well.

In the months leading up to winter, I advise you to take a more proactive stance - build up your child's immunity using essential oils. Should someone in the house be ill already, diffuse essential oils into the atmosphere to kill airborne bacteria and viruses.

Essential oils can be used not only to kill off existing bugs but also as a preventative treatment as well. Lavender oil used in a daily massage will help to boost immunity and kill off bugs before they get a foothold. When your child is 6 months or older, you can further boost immunity by adding the appropriate oils to your 's bath once or twice a week. Tea Tree oil is a very effective stimulant when it comes to the immune system. You can also mix up a batch of 5 drops of the oil in 50ml of any carrier oil or aqueous cream and massage into your baby's the bottom of your baby's feet or into the palms of your baby's hands once or twice a week.

Diffusing Tea Tree oil can help to boost your whole family's immunity. Diffuse in sessions of 15 minutes at a time daily for two-three weeks and then leave off it for a week again to give your baby's system a break.

If Tea Tree oils does not appeal to you, you can choose any of the following, once you baby is 6 months old or older:

Tea Tree oil, Basil oil, Lavender oil, Eucalyptus oil, Bergamot oil, Rosemary oil. Lavender oil can be used to boost immunity in this manner from the age of 10 weeks on.

## Immune Boosting Blend

(Suitable for ages 6 months and up)

2 drops Bergamot oil

2 drops Lavender oil

2 drops Sandalwood oil

60 ml carrier oil of your choice

Mix all the oils together and massage into baby's feet once or twice a week.

Alternatively, swap out the carrier oil for 125ml milk and halve the amount of essential oils and add to baby's bath water.

You can also skip the carrier oil altogether and use the oils in the diffuser.

# Immune Boosting Cream

(Suitable for ages 10 weeks and up)

2 drops Lavender oil

2 drops Chamomile oil

40ml aqueous cream

Mix all the oils together and massage into baby's feet once or twice a week.

Alternatively, swap out the carrier oil for 125ml milk and halve the amount of essential oils and add to baby's bath water.

You can also skip the carrier oil altogether and use the oils in the diffuser.

# Beating Anxiety

There is a very definite link between increased levels of anxiety and a higher risk of contracting an illness. Making sure that your baby is happy is just as essential when it comes to boosting their immune system as feeding them the right food is.

You can kick off this process by giving your baby a massage on a daily basis - alternate with your spouse if you need to but do make sure to have this time with baby on a regular basis - by doing the massage, you will be able to notice if something is wrong very quickly.

In addition to the massage, you should also make time to play with baby every day as well - quality learning time is an important part of baby's development and I very serious doubt that you will one day look back and say, "I wish I had not spent so much time with my baby."

Babies also pick up on the mood of their parents very quickly so if you are stressed about something, you need to try and deal with as quickly as possible. Essential oils can help with this as well. Here are some oils that you can use during play time with baby that will relax both of you.

## Sunshine Oil

(Suitable for ages 6 months and older)

1 Drops Neroli oil

1 Drops Lavender oil

1 Drops Ylang Ylang oil (Optional - omit if the scent does not appeal to you)

1 Drops Sandalwood oil

This blend is best used in a diffuser for the benefit of both you and your baby but you can also mix it into 40ml of either a carrier oil or an aqueous base of your choice and massage into skin and tight muscles to promote relaxation.

## Happy Baby

1 drop Bergamot oil

1 drop Sandalwood oil

1 drop Neroli oil

Place all the oils in a diffuser and use during playtime with baby to give both of you a mood boost.

# Sleepless Nights

Being tired can wear you down, you know this. If baby doesn't sleep well at night, his immune system will become weaker and he will be more likely to get ill. Using oils to calm baby before bedtime can help him to get a better night's rest and help him to make him full of energy the next day.

These blends can also help you get a more peaceful night's rest - while the saying goes that you should sleep like a baby, not many of us with small children actually aspire to that, especially not when baby wakes up every few hours.

Here are some blends that are great for those times when baby just cannot, or will not, fall asleep:

# Goodnight Baby Mix

(Suitable for ages 10 weeks and up)

1 drop Lavender oil

1 drop Chamomile oil

20ml carrier oil of your choice

Mix all ingredients and massage into back, chest and feet just before bedtime. The massage in itself can help to soothe your baby and the oils will make him sleepy.

# Sweet Dreams Mix

(Suitable for ages 6 months and up)

1 drops Chamomile oil

1 drops Ylang Ylang oil (Optional)

1 drops Lavender oil

1 drops Cedar Wood oil

80ml carrier oil of your choice

In this blend, the Ylang Ylang won't be too obvious so you don't need to worry about it upsetting the balance of the blend. When used in small amounts, it can be helpful at creating a feeling of contentment and relaxation.

Mix all the oils together and rub into the soles of baby's feet just before bed time.

If baby us suffering from sinusitis, this blend can help if you omit the Ylang Ylang and rub it into the back and neck.

It can also help to soothe dry skin if you swap out the oil for a rich aqueous cream.

# Conclusion

Thank you again for downloading this book!

I hope that you enjoyed reading this book and that you learned a lot that you can use at home to make your baby's life a happier and healthier one. I hope that you understand the role that essential oils can play as a very valid alternative therapy now and how you can use this to your advantage.

Essential oils changed my life for the better and I trust that they will do the same for you. All you really have left to do now is to go and experiment with making your own blends and that is really the fun part - go and play the mad scientist to your heart's content.

Consistency is key when it comes to benefiting from essential oils - you really only need to start using them on a regular basis to start reaping long-term benefits.

Just one last thing - I would really love to know what you thought about this book. Please let me know by posting a review on Amazon. That would really be amazing and I am looking forward to hearing from you.

Thank you and good luck!